forever weight loss ©

A Simple 10-Step Plan
to a Lighter and Happier You

"A very reasonable, hands-on plan, that gets results."

Dr. Joseph DiRenzo Jr.
Philadelphia College of
Osteopathic Medicine

I lost 60 Pounds & Kept it Off for over 6 Years!

Includes 70 Very Easy Recipes

Robert D'Agostino M.L.I.S.

Published by Hallard Press LLC.
www.HallardPress.com   Info@HallardPress.com   352-234-6099
Bulk copies of this book can be ordered at Info@HallardPress.com

Printed in the United States of America

ISBN: 978-1-951188-21-4

Disclaimer: The author is not a trained dietician, nutritionist, or
medical professional. The information in this book is based on facts,
research, and personal experiences. This information is not intended
to diagnose, prevent, treat or cure any disease. Never dismiss any
advice your health physician gives. The author shall in no event be
held liable for any loss or other damages including but not limited to
special, incidental, consequential, or any other damages.

I would like to offer a sincere thank you to my family, friends and acquaintances who have helped me with their guidance and encouragement.

Congratulations

For making this positive choice for yourself!

By following the Forever Weight-Loss Plan, you will lose extra weight for the long-term, so you won't have to yo-yo diet anymore. You will look and feel better, look younger, feel accomplished, increase your energy, reduce your aches and pains, help prevent disease and enjoy your life more!

I understand what you've been going through. I have experienced the same frustrations as you have, riding on that diet roller coaster that focuses on just short-term results.

NOW is the time for you to get off that crazy ride and join the many who have followed the **Forever Weight-Loss Plan** which focuses on long-term weight-loss, and who now enjoy feeling lighter and healthier each and every day.

You will never have to be on another weight-loss plan again. Losing extra weight and keeping it off is very possible when you learn some simple can-do strategies.

The first important strategy is to **never blame yourself.** Blaming yourself is a negative emotion that will just add more stress to your life and encourage you to eat more than you need to. It's understandable why many of us eat more than we should. It's mainly because there are just too many bad processed food temptations out there, everywhere we go.

By following the **Forever 10-Step Weight-Loss Plan,** you will learn how to push away those processed food temptations and substitute them with **REAL FOOD,** which is a lot easier to manage.

You might be thinking, why can't I just shrink my food portions and exercise more to lose weight. Well, you can try that, but for most of us, it's very difficult to do so, and who really wants to exercise much more than you need to. I will show you an **EASIER WAY.**

I will show you how to train your body to slowly need less food and be very satisfied at the same time.

I created a plan where you don't have to count calories, cook too much or shake your booty too hard. A plan that is easy and flexible. The Forever Weight-Loss Plan is about building a new relationship with real food for the long-term, it's that simple. It's a 10-Step weight-loss plan that really works.

Contents

#1 Acceptable Food List

INTRODUCTION

The main strategy I used to lose weight and keep it off for over six years now, was to slowly train my body to want or need less food by eliminating bad processed food temptations and cravings as much as possible. I accomplished this by creating and focusing on my own personal #1 Food List and Menu with real foods and simple meals that I enjoy.

If you focus on those foods and **meals that you enjoy and look forward to**, you will be much less tempted to indulge in those awfully addictive processed foods again.

The reason why we are so attracted to processed foods is because they are fairly inexpensive and convenient. That's the keyword, convenient. That's how they get us. For the most part, processed foods contain extra amounts of chemical additives, sugar, salt and fat which can become addictive. Do you think that most food manufacturers are interested in your health? I don't think so.

Most manufacturers design their products that way, so we keep coming back for more and help them make more money, but we can be smarter than that by rediscovering **real food** once again.

Remember, it's all about the types of food you eat, that determine the amount of food you eat; and the amount of food that you eat determines how heavy or light you want to be.

There are just 2 types of food out there; those that you can control and those that you can't! Most overweight folk eat food that they can't control. It's a lot easier to control real food than processed food.

When I was overweight, I had a hard time controlling donuts and ice cream. If you can't control certain foods, try your best to eliminate them from your personal menu for a while. By doing this, you will most likely lose your strong desire or craving for them, as I did.

I'm not saying you should eliminate them for the rest of your life, but just for a while, until you reach your desired weight. You will most likely lose your craving for large amounts of them anyhow and be satisfied with smaller portions instead.

I will show you how I lowered my food intake to about HALF of what I used to eat and continue to enjoy the foods I have always loved, except, I enjoy them in smaller portions.

Not because I choose to deny myself, but because I just do not need certain foods or desire larger portions anymore. I have successfully weaned myself away from those high-carb, high-sugar and high-fat foods, which only threatened my weight-loss goal and my health. It took me a little while to be completely satisfied with less, but I am so much happier that I did.

I now have a thinner body which feels great. Remember, a lighter body requires less food than a heavier body does.

It's all about finding quality foods that you look forward to eating. I now put more thought into all my meal choices. I first think about what I'm in the mood for, salty, sweet, savory, and then search for quality. No impulse buys for me.

I rely on my **personally designed menu and my #1 Food List to keep me on track.** By eating throughout the day, whenever I'm hungry, about every 2-3 hours and exercising on a slow, that's right, a slow routine basis, no crazy workouts for me; my body adjusted to needing less.

I now enjoy feeling much lighter and healthier than ever before and so will you, if you follow my **10-Step plan.**

The trick is to create simple, healthy convenience foods for yourself, so you won't be tempted by those bad processed food temptations anymore.

Why I got serious about losing weight?

Well, there were **three** reasons why I decided that it was time to make a positive change for myself and lose my extra weight.

The **first** reason was when my cousin told me one day, at a family gathering, that I looked fat. Whoa, wakeup call! I love my cousin and I know she loves me, but she could have been more politically correct and called me overweight, but honestly, it just wouldn't have had the same impact, would it?

It seemed hurtful at first, but it was true. Thank you, cousin Hilda for your tough love. So, when I returned home and compared my past photos with my current ones, I really noticed how much heavier I had become. Yuck!

I was actually 60 pounds heavier than I have ever been. Sixty pounds is a lot. That's 12 five-pound bags of sugar or flour.

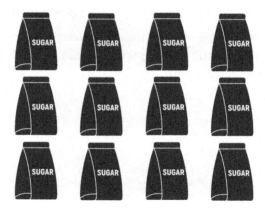

So, why wasn't it easy for me to look at myself in the mirror and admit that? Why was it so hard for me to admit that I needed to make a change? Why is it so hard for most of us to make a lifestyle change for ourselves?

It's because we get stuck in our **comfort zone.** You know the place. A place where you don't want change and just want to keep your stress and anxiety at a minimum. That's why. It's very surprising to know how much we will tolerate before we take the necessary steps to make a healthy change for ourselves. **So, don't blame yourself. You are not alone.**

The **second** reason for making a change was when I visited my doctor for my annual checkup. I told him that my eyes were blurry more often than not, and I was much more tired than usual. I thought I was just overworked. I was running a restaurant six nights a week and working full-time as a high school Librarian.

So, when my doctor came back with my blood results and told me that I was Type 2 diabetic, I couldn't believe it. I was both shocked and scared. I guess I was eating much more than I needed to. Most likely, I was eating too much of the wrong foods.

The **third** reason was that I just got fed-up with looking and feeling terrible. I just couldn't take it anymore. Every time I had to do the stairs, I had knee pain. Each night I went to bed, I snored heavily and had difficulty breathing, because I acquired sleep apnea.

I had back pain and low energy. My belly hung over my belt.

My thighs rubbed against each other. My clothes didn't fit right, and I didn't want to spend more money to bump up to a larger size once again. I couldn't even find the motivation to exercise anymore because I was carrying an extra 60 pounds on my body everywhere I went.

Finally, because of all these reasons, I decided to make a change for myself and commit to losing all those unwanted pounds.

I began to search for a weight-loss book that I could live with, one that would give me long-term, weight-loss results.

But after reviewing over 125 weight-loss books, I soon became very discouraged, because most weight-loss plans are too restrictive and designed just for the short term. So after much thought, I decided to create my own plan. A plan that really works.

So now is the time for you to invest in yourself and commit to losing all those unwanted pounds for the long-term because you are definitely worth it.

But before you start with the 10-steps, I would like you to complete your very own Treat List. A list of rewarding ways to treat yourself other than with food. Don't get me wrong, food is an important and enjoyable part of life, but it shouldn't be the only place to find comfort and gratification.

Treat List

1._____

2._____

3._____

4._____

5._____

6._____

7._____

8._____

9._____

10._____

Here are some of the ways I treat myself other than with food:

- **See a new movie or an old one again**
- **Go to a concert or play**
- **Hang out with friends or family**
- **Get a massage**
- **Visit a favorite place, close or far**
- **Buy myself something**
- **Take an enrichment class**
- **Go dancing**
- **Listen or sing to my favorite music**
- **Bring joy to someone else**
- **Share a smile or a hug**
- **Practice Yoga**

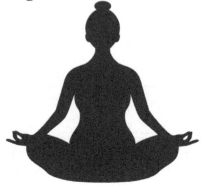

Chapter One

SHOP for kitchen items that will help you lose weight and keep it off.

STEP 1

- 20 oz bowl

WHY? Because eating from a bowl rather than a plate, subconsciously, helps you with portion control. Instead of having your servings piled high on a plate, you get portion control without even knowing it. A bowl is easier to carry and hold when watching TV or the computer.

- 1/3 clear measuring cup

The measuring cup is the exact amount of grain, pasta or starchy vegetable you can eat per day if you choose to.

- Small fork and teaspoon

WHY? Because they help you to eat slower by eating smaller portions at a time. When you eat slower, you slow down your rate of consumption which gives your stomach time to send a message to your brain that you're full and it's time to stop eating.

-     10-inch non-stick frying pan

The frying pan will cook your 1/3 cup of pasta or starchy vegetable and also be used to cook all of your meals.

-     8 oz. drinking cup
-     Cooking oil pump or spray

Remember, these are **your** kitchen items, you are cooking for one. Unless, of course, someone in your household wants to join you on your weight-loss journey.

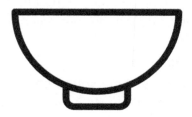

STEP 2

SELECT & HIGHLIGHT the foods that you like at the #1 Acceptable Food List form at ForeverWeightLossPlan.com.

WHY? If you narrow down your choices to the **REAL** foods that you like, it will be much easier for you to lose weight, because you will be taking a break from those heavily processed foods. It's all about being satisfied with smarter, real food choices, that you enjoy.

When you eat healthy foods that satisfy your appetite, you will automatically, without really thinking about it, consume fewer calories, and fewer calories mean less weight. The #1 Acceptable Food List will be your eating guide, so keep it with you on your phone or tablet. I was determined to lose the extra weight in a shorter period of time, so I stayed solely with my #1 Food List and my personally designed menu for over 12 months. You decide what works best for you.

LOVE REAL FOOD is the mantra. Now is the time to rediscover real food because you deserve the best, your body deserves the best and **you deserve to look and feel better.**

Remember, the longer you are able to stay away from those high-fat, high-sugar, and high-calorie foods, you will find that you will slowly lose your desire for them.

Now don't worry, I'm not asking you to eliminate all processed foods from your #1 list. There are some processed foods out there that are low in fat, sugar and calories that you can add to your list if you like.

But before you choose, you need to know how to read a nutrition label and know what you're really getting, because food labels can be tricky and deceptive.

Let's take sugar for example. In order for you to know the actual amount of sugar in a food item, you need to multiply the grams of sugar x the number of servings. This will equal the actual amount of sugar in a container.

Grams of sugar x servings = total amount of sugar.

Look at the food label and you will see that 6 grams of sugar is per serving, not per container. That's 6 servings x 6 grams of sugar. 6 x 6 = 36 grams of sugar.

There are 9 teaspoons of added sugar in that marinara sauce, because 4 grams of sugar = 1 teaspoon of sugar.

Marinara Sauce

Nutrition Facts
Serving Size: ½ cup
Servings per Container: 6

Amount per Serving
Calories: 80

Total Fat 1.5g	2%
Sodium 330 mg	16%
Total Carbohydrate 10g	3%
Dietary Fiber 1g	4%
Sugar 6g	
Protein 2g	

Vitamin A 8%	Vitamin C 10%
Calcium 2%	Orin 4%

Percent values are based on a 2,000 calorie diet.
Your Daily Values may be higher or lower depending
on your calorie needs.

INGREDIENTS: Tomato Puree (Water, Tomato
Paste), Diced Tomatoes, Sugar, Natural Oil Blend
(palm kernel, extra virgin olive oil and fish oil),
Celery, Onion, Salt, Garlic Powder, Onion Powder,
Spices, Citric Acid, Pectin, Natural Flavor, Vitamin E,
Vitamin B6

Nine teaspoons of sugar may not seem like much at first, but when you add all the other foods that have sugar in them for that day, you will see how it really adds up. Added sugar means added calories and added fat.

Now choose

A low carb tortilla brand

I chose Trader Joe's low-carb tortilla because they are the lowest carb bread product I could find, that I like.

Low carb bread products vary considerably both in taste and texture.

If you can find a low carb bread product that you like that is under 10 carbs per slice, then by all means make that your choice.

Eat only 2 low-carb tortillas or slices of bread per day, if you choose to.

They don't have to be wheat, but make sure they're under 10 carbs per tortilla.

After I lost my desired weight, I tried eating other types of bread again, but bread is very high in carbs and difficult for me to control, so I have stayed away from it. I don't miss bread much anymore because it makes me feel too full. I am now satisfied with just one slice of toasted sourdough bread with a little cream cheese and jelly in the morning.

Now choose

A pasta tomato sauce

Most sauces have a lot of sugar in them, so narrow down

your favorite choice that has the least amount. Sugar is just added calories which will make it much harder for you to lose weight and keep it off.

Now choose

Some condiments

There are hundreds of processed condiments available and most of them have lots of sugar in them. Find the ones that you like with the least amount of sugar. Condiments can be a life changer when it comes to food enjoyment, so choose wisely.

Ideally, you want to choose a condiment with no added sugar at all. If you find one, that's great. They're out there. Don't give up. Remember that added sugar is just added fat pounds for you.

Food manufacturers add sugar to most all processed foods. They even add sugar to meat products, watch out for that BBQ rib sauce. So why do they do this? Because sugar is addictive. They want you to keep coming back for more. You can't lose weight and keep it off if you have to have sugar in everything you eat. So, stay away from any tomato sauce or condiment that have more than 2 grams of sugar per serving.

Now choose

Your favorite drinks and enter them on your #1 food list.

Most drinks have a lot of sugar in them, so narrow down your favorites that have the least amount.

Sodas, juices and most tea and coffee drinks are full of sugar, which, as you know, just contain extra calories that will convert to fat. Instead, try an herbal tea that is naturally flavored that doesn't have sugar, like a chai or fruit tea. There are lots of them out there to choose from. Any added sugar, including honey, is just added calories that you do not need. A little sugar here and a little sugar there, just adds up to a lot of sugar in your body, which will convert to more added fat for you. Sodas and juices are not permitted on the #1 food list.

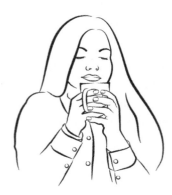

If you choose to drink tea or coffee drinks, make sure that they have less than 4 grams of sugar per drink. That's one teaspoon of sugar per drink. If you can, try to eventually cut that in half. Even this little change will make a huge difference in the long run.

Did you know that milk contains sugar? That's more unneeded calories for you. Only drink a little. Remember that 4 grams of sugar = 1 teaspoon of sugar.

Grams of sugar per cup of milk

7g oat
8g coconut

10g soy
12g skim
12g 2%
12g whole
12g lactose free
13g almond
13g 1%
13g rice

Before you choose your drinks, do at least one drink comparison and make the better choice for yourself.

WHY SHOULD I COMPARE DRINKS?

Because food and drink can be very deceiving. You might think that you are drinking for weight-loss, but after writing down their nutritional content, you are very likely to surprise yourself. Before I started on my plan, I didn't think I was really eating or drinking that much. Sure enough, I was consuming way too many calories, which included a lot of sugar and carbs. Focus on making better food and drink choices for yourself because **you deserve the best.**

You can save yourself many unnecessary calories, just by making the smarter drink choice. Look at this comparison.

VANILLA FRAPPUCCINO

430 Cal, 72g carbs, 71g sugar—that's 17.75 tsp of sugar

ICED CAFE MOCHA

350 Cal, 39g carbs, 30g sugar — that's 7.5 tsp of sugar

ICED CAFE LATTE

130 Cal, 13g carbs, 11g sugar — that's 2.75 tsp of sugar

Now complete your drink comparison

_____name ___ calories ___ carbs ___ sugar

_____name ___ calories ___ carbs ___ sugar

_____name ___ calories ___ carbs ___ sugar

_____name ___ calories ___ carbs ___ sugar

_____name ___ calories ___ carbs ___ sugar

How about water?

Yes, drinking water will help you lose weight. Water helps boost your metabolism, cleanses your body of waste, and acts as an appetite suppressant.

There is no set amount you should drink; drink when you're thirsty. I do suggest you drink at least 6 oz of water after you wake up in the morning. Your body has been without liquids for over 8 hours, so you should rehydrate first thing. It really helps with getting that waste out of your body.

Keeping your body hydrated at the start of the day, helps the blood flow to your skin, releases toxins and fat cell by-products from your system and protects your colon and bladder from infections, so drink water whenever you can.

STEP 3

DESIGN your own menu

This is the most important part of your weight-loss plan.

Don't forget, you're in charge. You decide what you put in your body. You have the power. Your goal is to feel satisfied with the food choices you list in your personally designed menu. Meal choices that you enjoy and look forward to.

Check out the many easy meal suggestions I created for you on pg. 59. If you have time to create more involved meals, there are of course thousands of cookbooks to choose from out there. I prefer easy and quick meal combinations.

Even though I was a former chef, I don't want to spend a lot of time in the kitchen preparing meals during my work week. I would rather create more elaborate meals on the weekends, when I have more time. I tried spaghetti squash in place of spaghetti once. Didn't like it much because it doesn't taste like pasta. I like pasta, always have, always will. Can't be replaced with thinly sliced squash. So, enjoy 1/3 cup of pasta if you really want to, **only once per day** that is.

Now create a list of meals for yourself using only foods from the #1 Acceptable Food List and the very easy recipes I created for you on pg. 59. Feel free to create and add your own recipes of course. Use the online form at ForeverWeightLossPlan.com—this can be fun.

WHY? Because, by having real foods readily available throughout the day, you won't be as tempted to make poor choices at the convenience store, vending machines or coffee shop. You will create a list of delicious, simple, and easy to make meals for yourself. This will be **your eating guide.**

How about snacks?

I don't define small amounts of food as snacks as the dictionary does. I would rather label snacks as meals, because a snack can, in many instances, contain as many calories as a full meal. So, do your best to **have something prepared and available for yourself every 2-3 hours each day. Create your own convenience food.**

When you create your own food menu, you won't be as tempted to impulsively choose from other people's menus, which will only sidetrack your weight-loss goal. Your meals should be what you like, what you are in the mood for and what will satisfy you. You decide. **You're the boss. You're in charge. It's really all about you, because it's your weight-loss goal that matters.**

What do I do when I visit a restaurant?

That's easy. Just open your menu on your smartphone or tablet wherever you go and let your online menu and food list be your guide. If you really have to have some bread with your meals, bring your low-carb tortillas with you in the car.

I bought a small, inexpensive cooler for my car that I plug in to my charging port. I bring my tortillas with me sometimes if I'm eating out locally or when I'm travelling. Sounds a little extreme. Not at all, if you're really serious about losing weight and keeping it off, almost nothing's extreme.

STEP 4

LIST the processed foods and drinks that you CRAVE that are **not** on your #1 food list.

I mean, the food and drinks that you cannot control. If you were lying on your deathbed, ask yourself which foods you would really regret not eating more of. I suspect that eating more processed foods wouldn't be one of your regrets. I know it wouldn't be for me. There are many more important things in life than eating more addictive processed foods.

Donuts and ice cream were my addiction. I can't eat donuts anymore because I can't digest the bad processed oil they cook them in or the highly processed sugar they add, which is much too sweet for me now. Same goes with ice cream. Even the quality brands have become too sweet for me. If I have any, I'll look for a high-quality brand and satisfy myself with just a little.

Once you have completed your food craving list, you can choose only 1 item from this list to eat during each week, if you really need to. I call this a transition or cheat food. Choose and enter it on your #1 Acceptable Food List only if you really need to. **I understand it isn't easy** to transition from your old menu to your new one, so this step will help you, only if you really need to. Not in a good way, but in a necessary way for a very, very short period of time.

Remember to only choose one of the same item per week. Donuts one-week, fried chicken the next, only if you really need to, because eating these foods will only make it that much harder for you to lose weight and keep it off.

I was a donut eater, but when I completed a nutrition checklist, I really saw what I was putting in my body and I was shocked.

Eating 1 **DONUT** a day isn't that bad, but who can only eat one. That's because donuts can be addictive, not unlike any other sugary, processed food. I weaned myself to two donuts a day, then one, then none. As I began to eat more real food, **processed food began to make me sick,** so I wasn't tempted by them anymore. You should find that too.

1 DONUT

CALORIES	320
FAT	(15) grams
CARBS	43 grams
SUGAR	22 grams = 5 ½ teaspoons sugar

2 DONUTS

CALORIES	640
FAT	(30) grams
CARBS	86 grams
SUGAR	44 grams = 11 teaspoons sugar

3 DONUTS

CALORIES	(960)
FAT	45 grams
CARBS	129 grams
SUGAR	66 grams = 16 1/2 teaspoons sugar

Now take some time to really think about this, and then enter the sugar, carb and calorie content of each, so you can really see what you are putting in your body. Visit an online calorie counter do this.

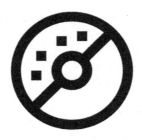

Now list all of your processed and/or your deep fried food cravings and nutritional content

_____name ___ calories ___ carbs ___ sugar

_____name ___ calories ___ carbs ___ sugar

_____name ___ calories ___ carbs ___ sugar

_____name ___ calories ___ carbs ___ sugar

_____name ___ calories ___ carbs ___ sugar

_____name ___ calories ___ carbs ___ sugar

_____name ___ calories ___ carbs ___ sugar

_____name ___ calories ___ carbs ___ sugar

STEP 5

CREATE your food shopping list

Make an online shopping list of the foods you need and enjoy for the meals you have created for yourself. Visit **ForeverWeightLossPlan.com** for a shopping list form.

WHY? Because if you have all the food you need for the week, you won't be tempted to buy those heavily processed, high-calorie, high-fat foods from other places that will only threaten your weight-loss goal.

Remember, whatever you decide to bring into your house, apt or workplace is key to losing weight and keeping it off. If a pint of ice cream is in my house, I will finish it, most likely in one sitting. If I bring in a bag of chocolate, I will finish it. I know which foods I can't control, so I keep my distance from them.

If I do bring in a pint of ice cream in my house, which I rarely do, I will make sure others in my household want some too. This is a good strategy after you have lost all your desired weight first. If you buy something you can't control, make sure you have others who will share it with you.

STEP 6

PURGE your processed foods

Purge your home, car and workplace of all processed foods. I know this won't be easy at first, especially if you have a partner, a spouse or a family that you live with, **but it needs to be done.** No processed, no temptation.

Also, set aside a space for yourself in a cupboard, the refrigerator and the freezer. You are a VIP, a very important person, with a mission. Don't forget that. You deserve your own space. Do not allow anyone to sidetrack your weight-loss goal. **You are doing great so far.**

WHY? Because eating highly processed foods will NOT help you lose weight and keep it off. Donate or discard them. Most highly processed food manufacturers design their products specifically just to get you hooked.

STEP 7

SHOP for REAL FOOD

Visit your favorite places to food shop. But keep in mind, that most foods sold at supermarkets are highly processed, so stick to your online food list.

Have you visited a local food co-op or health food store lately? Both can be fun places to shop, but not unlike your local market, they also have many high-sugar, high-carb and high-calorie foods on the shelf, so be wary.

Just because it's a health food store, or food co-op, it doesn't mean that everything in the store is healthy for you, so remember to stay with your list.

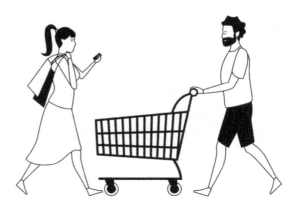

STEP 8

EAT and ENJOY

Satisfy yourself by grazing on real food throughout the day. I suggest every 2-3 hours. I say this, because this will help keep your blood sugar level and help you slowly lose your unhealthy cravings. Of course, you're not going to lose all of your cravings entirely at first. Some cravings will take longer than others. **That's understandable.**

Before you choose something to eat, ask yourself, what am I in the mood for? Do I feel like something savory, salty, sweet or crunchy? Most of us do that without really thinking about it, but now I am asking you to think about it before you choose. Listen first, choose second, eat third.

Once you start to eat REAL FOOD again, you will begin to appreciate how delicious real food can be.

I think a lot of us back off from fresh foods because we think it takes too much time to

make quick and easy meals with them, but this is not true.

I devote just 20-40 minutes each weekend to prepare vegetables, meat, fish and some wild rice for the week. Because I prepare these foods in advance, all I have to do is assemble them and heat them up during the work week.

It's such a good feeling to open the fridge and have all the real foods that I like, already prepared for me, whenever I'm hungry.

I don't cook pasta and potatoes ahead of time because I end up eating more than I need at one sitting. So, cook 1/3 cup to order only once per day if you're in the mood. Use your 10 inch frying pan to boil some water for your pasta.

Take a look at all the quick and easy wraps and dishes I created for you on page 59. There are hundreds of quick and easy real food combinations out there that you can make. Believe me.

When should I eat?

You should eat when you're hungry. That's it. No restrictive schedule to follow.

It's not about eating at preset times of the day, like you have been doing in the past. You are retraining your body to only eat when you are actually hungry, not because the clock, your friends, your relatives, the government, or anybody else for that matter should tell you when or what you should eat.

You eat what you like, when you like, as long as your choices are from your #1 Acceptable Food List.

Listen to your stomach and eat when you are hungry; it does speak to you. It's ok to be hungry. After a period of time, you just won't desire large meals anymore, because by grazing, every 2-3 hours, throughout the day, you will find satisfaction, you will find contentment.

The key to long term weight control is training your body to need less.

How many Calories should I eat per day?

Calories do count of course, but we don't count them on the Forever Weight-Loss Plan. What a relief! You have better things to do with your time. Instead, focus on your MENU.

- **If you're hungry, go to your menu.**
- **Make sure you have food available at all times.**
- **Always replenish your food inventory, in the car, at work and at home.**

DO

- Be easy on yourself at all times
- Eat when you are hungry and eat quality
- Make fruit your sweet
- Make low-carb tortillas, or slices of bread, your bread choice for a while—only 2 per day if you want.
- Only eat 1/3 cup of pasta, rice or starchy vegetable only once per day if you choose to. If you want beans and rice, they should equal only 1/3 cup combined.
- Fill up with more non-starchy vegetables than with starchy ones. Look at the #1 Acceptable Food List.

DON'T

• Eat bakery products, other than the low-carb tortillas or slices of bread.

• Eat fried foods. They're not on the #1 Acceptable Food List. All oils, both healthy and not, are still 120 calories per tablespoon. That's a lot of unnecessary calories and fat. Use the oil pump or spray and sauté instead. Any food, deep fried, soaks up lots of oil. Oil is fat. Just take a look this comparison.

Look at this comparison:

FRIED

CHICKEN	FAT	CALORIES
1 Breast	18	423
1 Wing	7.25	102
1 Drumstick	6.8	119
TOTAL	**32 g**	**644**

BAKED

CHICKEN	FAT	CALORIES
1 Breast	3.6	165
1 Wing	2	42
1 Drumstick	2.5	76
TOTAL	**8.1 g**	**283**

STEP 9

SHAKE YOUR BOOTY in a small way, when you can

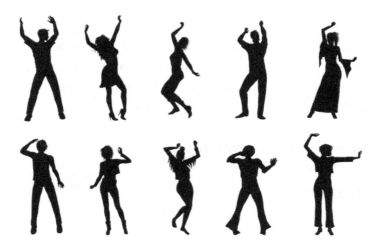

You can't lose weight and keep it off unless you move your body in some way almost every day. It doesn't have to be a timed regime at the gym. It doesn't have to be scheduled. It doesn't have to be hard. It just has to be done in some way, **every day.**

You might ask, why can't I just exercise every other day. Well, it's actually harder to do that, because most of us find it harder to keep track of and it's easier to find excuses.

You want to find physical activities that you like best and look forward to. The best way to stick with new, good habits for yourself, is to do them each day. The trick is not to think about it too much, just do it. Otherwise you will just talk yourself out of it.

I enjoy watching TV that I placed in front of my stationary bike for between 25 - 45 minutes each day. I also enjoy walking and riding my bike when it's nice out and climbing some stairs at my workplace before, after or during lunch each day. I also attend a yoga class once a week to maintain and improve my balance, flexibility, and muscle strength.

Please keep in mind that exercise isn't just for weight loss. It can benefit you in so many other ways. I lost about 60% of my extra weight on a slow daily basis and then I increased my routine to lose the other 30%. I am still working on the last 10%. Remember it's about progress not perfection. Believe me. Just move each day doing something that you enjoy. You won't be motivated to do it, if you don't enjoy it. Exercise is great for your mental well-being, and feeling good will help you stay on track with your weight-loss goal. Remember that exercise alone will never be enough to lose a lot of weight, unless you do a TON of it. **That's why it's all about the food that you choose to eat that's so important, so stick to your menu.**

Have you ever noticed how good you feel after a brisk walk, a swim, a bike ride or a jog? It's the release of endorphins and dopamine, the happy chemicals and the reduction in the stress hormones cortisol and adrenaline that make you feel so good. According to research, just 20 minutes of some type of exercise can boost your mood for up to 12 hours, so Walk, Bike, Garden, Dance, or practice Yoga when you can.

Once you start losing those extra pounds, you will be more motivated to exercise a little more each day, because you will have less pounds to carry around.

Now Create your own Booty Shaker list

1._____

2._____

3._____

4._____

5._____

STEP 10

GET HIGH the Natural Way

by activating your body's own natural, happy chemicals:

Dopamine, Serotonin, Endorphins and Oxytocin. You don't need those high-carb, sugary processed foods to do this. They will only satisfy your chemical need for a very short time and set you up for unhealthy food addiction. So try these much healthier ways to get your natural high.

Let's start with **Dopamine**. Dopamine is the hormone triggered when we approach and anticipate a reward and is associated with euphoria and bliss — hence its nickname "the feel-good hormone." When dopamine is released in the brain, you will get a good feeling accompanied by a surge of energy so you can realize that reward.

Dopamine motivates us to take action toward goals, desires, and needs, and gives a surge of reinforcing pleasure when achieving them.

Rather than only allowing our brains to celebrate when we've hit the finish line, you can create a series of little finish lines like the steps listed in this book. Don't forget to congratulate yourself and celebrate each time you complete a step.

You are doing great! Congratulations on your accomplishments so far.

The second feel good hormone is **Serotonin.** Serotonin is an important neurotransmitter in our body. It contributes to feelings of well-being and happiness. Serotonin flows when you feel significant or important. Loneliness and depression appear when serotonin is absent.

A popular way to boost your level of serotonin is by practicing gratitude. **Gratitude** for what you have now and what you have accomplished in the past. They remind us that we are valued and have much to value in life.

Gratitude is a gift we give to ourselves!

Now Create your Gratitude List

1._____

2._____

3._____

4._____

5._____

6._____

7._____

8._____

9._____

10._____

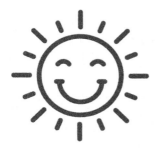

If you need a serotonin boost during the day, expose yourself to **natural daylight** for 20 minutes or more. Natural daylight promotes vitamin D and serotonin production in our bodies. I use a natural daylight lamp at my work desk and at home during wintertime.

The third feel good hormone are **Endorphins.** Endorphins are chemicals produced naturally by the nervous system.

Endorphins are released in response to pain and stress and help to alleviate anxiety and depression. The surging "second wind" and euphoric "runners high" during and after a vigorous run are a result of endorphins. Similar to morphine, it diminishes our perception of pain.

Instead of running laps to get your endorphin rush, why not try **laughter.** Yes laughter.

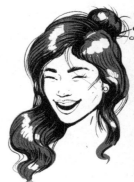

Even the anticipation of laugher increases our levels of endorphins. Taking your sense of humor to work, forwarding that funny email, and finding several things to laugh at during the day is a great way to keep the doctor away.

And the fourth and last feel-good natural hormone is **oxytocin.** Oxytocin is also sometimes referred to as the "love hormone," because levels of oxytocin increase during hugging and orgasm. It may also have benefits as a treatment for a number of conditions, including depression and anxiety.

Oxytocin creates intimacy, trust, and builds healthy relationships. It's released by men and women during orgasm, and by mothers during childbirth and breastfeeding. Animals will reject their offspring when the release of oxytocin is blocked.

The cultivation of oxytocin is essential for creating strong bonds and improved social interactions. Often referred to as the cuddle hormone, a simple way to keep oxytocin flowing in your body is to simply, give someone **a hug.**

Inter-personal touch not only raises oxytocin but reduces cardiovascular stress and improves the immune system; so rather than just a handshake, go in for the hug, if it's ok with the person you want to hug. Dopamine, serotonin, oxytocin and endorphins is the quartet responsible for a lot of our happiness.

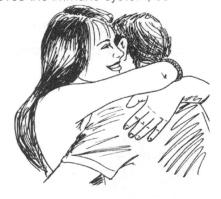

Try your best to find those things that redirect you away from food as a primary source of comfort.

Sure, I get stressed, bored and lonely at times, but I deal with these stressors in more positive ways. There are many joys out there, it's just a matter of rediscovering them. So, for a happy, no calorie hormone boost, try smiling, laughing, touching, or singing and listening to your favorite music.

SMILING

Can improve your mood

Even fake ones do the trick

Helps reduce stress

Makes you more approachable

Makes you seem more trustworthy

Retrains your brain for the better

Boosts your productivity

Strengthens the body on a cellular level

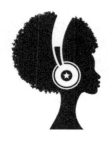

LISTENING to MUSIC

1. **Music increases Happiness.**
It only takes 15 minutes of listening to your favorite tunes to get a natural high. This is because our brain releases dopamine that leads to increased feelings of happiness, excitement, and joy.

2. Music Decreases Stress While Increasing Overall Health

Music decreases levels of the hormone cortisol in your body, **counteracting the effects of chronic stress**. Stress causes 60% of all illnesses and diseases, so lower levels of stress mean higher chances of overall well-being.

3. Music Improves Sleep

Over 30% of Americans suffer from insomnia. A study showed that listening to relaxing music within an hour of going to bed **significantly improves sleep.**

4. Music Reduces Depression

Music has a direct effect on our hormones; it can even be considered a natural antidepressant. This is because certain tunes cause the release of serotonin and dopamine in the brain which leads to increased feelings of happiness and well-being.

5. Music Helps You Eat Less

According to research, the combination of soft lighting and music leads people to **consume less food** and enjoy it more.

SINGING

Releases the same **feel-good** brain chemicals as sex and

chocolate! Singing is also very effective as a stress and pain reliever and just makes you feel great.

Now create your own Natural High list

1._____

2._____

3._____

4._____

5._____

6._____

7._____

8._____

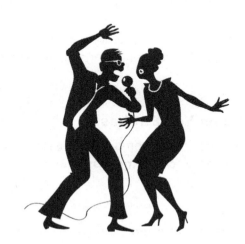

Chapter 2

CHOCOLATE

I have to talk about chocolate because most of us love chocolate, myself included. On average, each American consumes about twelve pounds of chocolate per year. That's much too much of course. We sometimes forget that the chocolate we eat is still **CANDY.** Most chocolate contains lots of sugar and lots of calories. If you can control your chocolate, then have a little. If you can't, do not include it on your #1 food list.

If you decide to buy some chocolate, always buy quality. A top quality chocolate product has cocoa as the first ingredient. Try to stay away from chocolate that has sugar as the first ingredient.

You have been told that chocolate has antioxidants, which are supposed to be healthy for you. Yes, that's true, but you have to consume the darkest chocolate with the least amount of sugar or milk to get any benefit at all. Keep in mind, that there are many other foods, such as delicious fruit, that contain antioxidants, which are much healthier for you with much less calories and fat.

If you want the benefits of chocolate without all the calories, consider making hot cocoa with a little sugar. Make sure to always choose quality. If you do need some chocolate, buy some and share some. You get your sweet fix and you feel good about sharing and make others happy too.

SUGAR baby, it's all the same.

I told my daughter that she has a sweet tooth because she loves sweets. She then told me, no Papa, all my teeth are sweet.

No matter what type you choose, sugar is sugar. Sugar is the generic name for sweet-tasting carbohydrates. Some sugars are more processed than others. Some are disguised as sugar. Take a look at the 56 forms of sugar.

1. Agave nectar
2. Barbados sugar
3. Barley malt,
4. Beet sugar
5. Blackstrap molasses
6. Cane sugar
7. Caramel
8. Carob syrup
9. Castor sugar
10. Confectioner's sugar
11. Corn syrup
12. Corn syrup solids
13. Crystalline fructose
14. Date sugar
15. Demerara sugar
16. Dextran
17. Dextrose
18. Diastatic malt
19. Diatase
20. Ethyl maltol

21. Evaporated cane juice
22. Florida crystals
23. Fructose
24. Fruit juice
25. Fruit juice concentrate
26. Galactose
27. Glucose
28. Brown rice syrup
29. Brown sugar
30. Buttered syrup
31. Cane juice crystals
32. Glucose solids
33. Golden sugar
34. Golden syrup
35. Grape sugar
36. High-fructose corn syrup
37. Honey
38. Icing sugar
39. Invert sugar
40. Lactose
41. Malt syrup
42. Maltose
43. Maple syrup
44. Molasses
45. Muscovado sugar
46. Organic raw sugar
47. Panocha
48. Raw sugar
49. Refiner's syrup
50. Rice syrup
51. Sorghum syrup
52. Sucrose
53. Sugar
54. Treacle
55. Turbinado sugar
56. Yellow sugar

Sugar is quick energy with lots of empty calories and added fat. In nature, sugars almost always come packaged with fiber, which slows their absorption rate and gives you a sense of fullness before you've ingested too many calories. That's why you're better off eating the fruit rather than drinking the juice, which is mostly sugar.

Unfortunately, processed sugar is in just about everything that is offered at the market. Why, because it tastes good, gives us a little rush and food manufactures know it can get us hooked. Sugar causes the release of the hormone dopamine in the brain, the same response activated by addictive drugs.

It's hard to live without some sugar, I know. **It's not easy for most of us.** I don't see myself not eating sugar anymore, so I've trained myself to be satisfied with less, by eating foods with natural sugars, such as fruit, vegetables and flavorful herbal teas, which are not addictive. If you can slowly wean yourself away from processed sugar, which I have, you will remove the need to eat most processed foods and **keep the extra weight off forever.**

When was the last time you heard of anyone addicted to fruit?

What about artificial sugar?

Well, artificial sugar is just that, artificial. I prefer not to put anything artificial in my body. If you use artificial sugars, I ask you first to taste the artificial sugar by itself first, before you add it to your food. Taste it and then decide if you really like artificial sugar.

How about ALCOHOL?

Alcoholic beverages are often high in empty calories and do not provide any real nutrients. Alcohol contains more calories per ounce than carbohydrates, because alcohol is made from sugar and starch.

Alcohol contains lots of calories; seven calories a gram in fact, almost as many as pure fat! As you well know, drinking alcohol just encourages us to eat more food (the munchies) and drink more alcohol than we planned. If you drink one glass of wine or one beer with your late afternoon or evening meal, that's fine, but remember that a lot of us drink for the buzz. The buzz usually makes us eat and drink more than we need, so if you really want to lose weight and keep it off, limit your alcohol.

FIBER helped me lose weight

Yes, eating foods that are fiber rich will help you lose weight because you will fill up quicker with foods that are mostly low in calories.

Fruits, vegetables, and whole grains contain ample amounts of fiber which will speed up your digestive system and get rid of your toxins and help you lose weight. You know how it feels when you release your poo. If it's done right, you actually feel lighter and much more relaxed.

But I found it difficult to eat enough natural fiber to be effective, especially when I'm trying to lose weight by eating less carbs.

Fortunately, I found another way. I found a fiber pill, namely the over the counter brand Metamucil or a generic brand, which contain Psyllium, a natural, soluble fiber. This natural fiber expands to form a gel-like substance in the gut, which has helped me feel fuller for longer and **helped me lose weight.** Psyllium is a relatively inexpensive, readily available source of fiber. It works wonders. I have been using it for six years now.

Please consult with your health physician first before you try a fiber pill.

In addition to fiber, another way to improve your digestion and lose weight, is to limit the size of your drinks with your meals. Drinking a full glass of milk, water, or alcohol with meals inhibits proper digestion and will make you feel full only for the short term because you are filling up with liquid.

Limit excessive drinking with your meals and you will stop diluting your digestive enzymes which are so important for proper digestion and weight loss.

70 VERY EASY RECIPES

I've listed some chef inspired meals for you

Simple recipes with no measurements, except for the 1/3 cup of pasta, rice or starchy vegetable, only if you want some.

If you minimize your starch carb, it will be much easier for you to lose weight and keep it off. Add more protein and/or non-starchy vegetables instead.

Just look at all the choices you have!

Remember that these recipes are very flexible, **YOU DECIDE** on the amount of each ingredient and how it is seasoned. **You are the boss. You are the chef.**

Visit **ForeverWeightLossPlan.com** for new recipes.

WRAPS

There are hundreds of delicious wrap combinations you can make. Who said that you have to eat processed? There are plenty of real food choices out there to satisfy your appetite.

SEAFOOD

- Salmon, grilled, baked or sautéed, mayo, lettuce
- Salmon smoked, cream cheese, red onion
- Shrimp summer roll, cold shrimp, basil leaves, julienned cabbage, carrot and cucumber, peanut sauce
- Crab salad
- Tuna melt, canned tuna, tomato, onion, mayo, cheese
- Tuna salad, canned tuna, celery, onion, mayo, shredded lettuce.

MEAT

- California club, fresh sliced chicken breast, crispy bacon, onion, mayo or Greek yogurt, avocado
- Chicken, feta, sun dried tomatoes, spinach
- Roast beef, horseradish, pepper jack cheese, melted
- Steak grilled, soy or steak sauce, guacamole, Pico de Gallo
- BLT, lean bacon, mayo, fresh tomato, lettuce
- Chicken breast grilled or blackened, lettuce, tomato, onions,

mayo or Greek yogurt

- Gyro, grilled lamb sausage, chopped lettuce, red onion, tomato, feta, Tzatziki sauce, cilantro, cucumber
- Chicken breast grilled or sautéed, avocado, onion, chopped tomatoes, Montery Jack cheese
- Chicken salad
- Pulled Pork, provolone, thinly sliced apples, kale, coleslaw
- Italian sausage, American and/or provolone cheese, sauteed onions, red and yellow peppers
- Reuben, real turkey, coleslaw, swiss cheese, sauerkraut, Russian dressing
- Asian chicken breast, soy, chopped roasted peanuts, cilantro, chile sauce, chopped green onions, coleslaw
- Ham and cheese
- Chicken or turkey, curry sauce, field greens, red onion, tomato
- Roast beef, onion, horseradish, mayo, arugula, tomato
- BBQ chicken
- Steak fajitas, roasted red & yellow peppers, onions
- Corned beef, sauerkraut, 1000 island dressing, Swiss cheese
- Buffalo chicken, hot sauce, cheddar cheese, tomato, onion
- Mu Shu pork, scrambled eggs, mushrooms, green onions, hoisin sauce
- Fresh turkey, tomato, mayo, onions, cranberry sauce, cheddar cheese

- Fresh turkey, avocado, tomato, onion
- Tacos, lean ground beef, lettuce, tomato, onion, hot sauce
- Cubano, roasted pork, ham, pickles, cheese of your choice
- Chorizo, egg and cheese

VEGE & others

- Hummus, sliced cucumber, tomato, sprouts
- PB&J
- Cheddar cheese, arugula, mayo
- Cheddar cheese and strawberry jelly
- Avocado, chopped tomato, hard-boiled egg
- The Greek, spinach, romaine, feta cheese, tomatoes, onion, Kalamata olives, Greek yogurt
- Egg and cheese, your way
- Portobello mushrooms, spinach, cheese, garlic
- Banana peppers, roasted, garlic, cheese
- Grilled corn, avocado, balsamic vinaigrette, roasted peppers
- Caprese, mozzarella, fresh basil, sliced tomato, olive oil
- Egg salad
- Tomato, vine-ripened, salt, mayo
- Guacamole
- Blackened fish, lettuce, tartar sauce, Cole slaw, fresh tomato

DISHES

VEGE

- Eggplant Parm, grilled, roasted or steamed, tomato sauce, mozzarella, grated Romano cheese
- Pesto, sautéed mushrooms, broccoli, 1/3 cup pasta
- Mushrooms, garlic, olive oil, broccoli rabe, a little cream cheese or Greek yogurt
- Cucumbers diced, tzatziki sauce, chopped peanuts
- Cauliflower + broccoli mashed, garlic, butter, salt
- Zucchini lasagna, steamed, thinly sliced zucchini, ricotta cheese, pasta sauce, some Romano or parmesan cheese and mozzarella. Melt together.
- Brussel sprouts, steamed then sautéed, garlic, olive oil, 1/3 cup rice
- Cole slaw

MEAT

- Steak grilled, 1/3 cup sweet potato, mushrooms, asparagus, garlic, olive oil
- Lamb grilled, green peas, cauliflower, asparagus, garlic, olive oil, Greek yogurt, 1/3 cup rice
- Chicken grilled, chopped tomatoes, chopped basil, mozzarella, a little parmesan, 1/3 cup rice

- Philly cheese steak, onions, red and yellow peppers, mushrooms, cheese of choice

SEAFOOD

- Shrimp sautéed with Bok choy, garlic, olive oil, 1/3 cup rice or pasta
- Flounder sautéed, baked or steamed, string beans, soy sauce, garlic, olive oil, 1/3 cup rice
- Salmon grilled, cauliflower, broccoli, julienned carrots, lemon butter sauce
- Coconut curry shrimp, red and yellow peppers, chopped peanuts, fresh basil leaf, bamboo shoots, curry sauce
- Shrimp steamed, chile sauce, ginger soy sauce, snow peas, 1/3 cup cooked rice

SOUP

- Thai Coconut soup from a can, mushrooms, shrimp, bamboo shoots, 1/3 cup rice
- Seafood chowder

CHAPTER 3

CONCLUSION...

If you really want to lose your extra weight and keep it off forever
stop **right here and stay with your #1 Food List and your personally designed menu.**

Jumping back into eating processed foods again will only frustrate you. It will set you up for sugar addiction and give you lots of unneeded stress and pounds. **Be easy on yourself. You deserve the best.**

You have accomplished so much, and **you should be very proud. Don't give up now.**

There is much more to enjoy in life than processed foods.

I'm still on the **Forever Weight-Loss Plan** and will be for the rest of my life, because it works. It has become a daily ritual, just like brushing my teeth. My personal menu will always be my guide.

But now, I don't need my food list anymore. The way I eat now has become second nature to me. I know what is best for me. I have lost my desire for those sugary, salty and fatty processed foods and I don't want to put those harmful foods in my body anymore. Now and then I might try one, but they will usually make me sick, because my body is now used to eating **REAL** food.

I've lost 60 pounds and I've kept them off for over 6 years now and have eliminated all my cravings. I am very proud of myself. Proud of losing my extra weight and keeping it off. I now eat whatever and whenever I want, but I eat smaller portions, not because I have to, but because I am satisfied with less.

I eat quality food in smaller portions throughout the day, and one larger, late afternoon meal. I am very happy that I created this new way of eating for myself and for you. **I deserve to feel great and so do you!** Now remember what I told you earlier in the book, that I was still working on the last 10% of my weight-loss goal. Sometimes I will gain a little weight now and then, called BUFFER WEIGHT, usually during the winter and I will lose it in the spring. It's understandable and I don't take it too seriously. I take it in stride and so should you.

Be easy on yourself. It's about progress, not perfection. Tomorrow is another day and **another chance for you** to feel better, healthier and lighter. **There is nothing that feels better than feeling lighter every day.**

MY DRINK COMPARISON

	carbs	calories	sugar	fat
ICED CAFE MOCHA	39	350	30	6
ICED SKINNY MOCHA	17	120	8	1.5

I chose the Iced Skinny Mocha of course. I don't need all those extra carbs, calories, sugar and fat. I made the better choice.

MY FOOD CRAVINGS

AMT	FOOD	Carbs	Calories	Sugar	Fat
1 PINT	HAAGEN DAZS ICE CREAM	77	910	70	60
1 DONUT		43	320	22	15
1 LARGE FRENCH FRIES		64	480	1	23

MY FOOD SHOPPING LIST

DAIRY	VEGES	FRUIT	MEAT FISH	CONDIMENTS
Milk non-fat	Eggplant	Watermelon	Clam	Mayo
Goat chs.	Mushroom	Cantaloupe	Mahi Mahi	Guacamole
Cream chs.	Squash	Grape	Steak	Salsa
Mozzarella	Onion	Cherry	Salmon	Pico de gallo
Cheddar	Jalapeno	Avocado	Duck	Cranberry Sauce
Romano	Romaine	Fig	Flounder	BBQ sauce
Greek Yogurt	Pepper	Honeydew	Lamb	Curry sauce
Ricotta	Asparagus	Nectarine	Oyster	Remoulade
Butter	Arugula	Peach	Turkey	Mustard
Swiss cheese	Cucumber	Pear	Pork	Ketchup
Sour cream	Celery	Apple	Tuna	Tzatziki sauce
Monterey Jack	Tomatoes	Blueberry	Haddock	Tartar sauce
Gorgonzola	Spinach	Mango	Chicken	Tomato sauce
American chs.	Bok Choy	Kiwi	Crab	Peanut sauce

MY GRATITUDE LIST

I AM GRATEFUL

That I caught my Type 2 diabetes just in time, before it got worse

For my overall good health

That I can find laughter in the world

For loving and enjoying many types of music

That I have people I care for and who care for me

For the sun and all the brightness and warmth that it brings

For my enthusiasm for learning

For my love of creativity

MY NATURAL HIGH LIST

Laughter

I watch SNL, and reruns of Seinfeld and Mad TV, and share jokes whenever I can.

Gratitude

Each morning I rise from bed, it's a birthday. My sunrise clock slowly brightens, and I awake. I stretch, practice some yoga and get ready for the day.

Smiling

After I wash my face in the morning, I smile in the mirror, well not really a smile, but rather a grin, like a cat. Not a creepy cat, but a curious and clever one.

Listening

I play music whenever and wherever I can.

Pet

My cat

Hug

My daughters

Singing and Dancing

At home and at work

Get some sun everyday it's shining

MY BOOTY SHAKER LIST

Bike riding
Yoga
Stationary bike
Walk outside
Climb stairs
Garden
Dance
Hike

PROCESSED FOOD INFO

Processed foods, such as ready meals, baked goods, and processed meats, can have negative health effects. Most food needs some degree of processing, and not all processed foods are bad for the body.

However, chemically processed foods, also called ultra-processed foods, tend to be high in sugar, artificial ingredients, refined carbohydrates, and trans-fats. Because of this, they are a major contributor to obesity and illness around the world.

Trans-Fat

When a regular fat like corn, soybean, or palm oil is blasted with hydrogen and turned into a solid, it becomes a trans-fat. Stay away from any food that lists shortening or partially hydrogenated oil as an ingredient. Labels boasting "zero trans- fat" don't always mean a food is completely trans-fat free. By law (FDA), such foods can contain 0.5 grams of trans-fats per serving. Trans-fat is bad for your heart and your waistline. Avoid fried foods from most restaurants and vendors since they most always use trans-fats to cook your food in. It's worth asking them what type of cooking oil they do use.

High Fructose Corn Syrup

According to researchers at Tufts University, Americans consume more calories from high fructose corn syrup than any other source. It's in practically EVERYTHING we eat and drink. It boosts fat-storing hormones, and drives people to overeat and gain weight. Any food that has been canned, dehydrated, or had chemicals added to it, is a processed food, and these foods make up about 70 percent of the average American diet. Avoid eating foods that list more than five or six ingredients.

Also, be aware of the many phrases manufacturers use on food products to capture our attention and persuade us to buy their product. Take a look at some of the most common deceptive food claims.

All Natural

Unfortunately, the FDA doesn't have an official definition for natural foods. That means there's room for interpretation. Seeing the word "natural" on a food product may not mean what you hope it means. Without any formal regulation, the consumer is left to trust the food manufacturers. A food product that's made with "all-natural" ingredients could still contain hormones, GMOs, or other things some consumers worry about. All-natural foods can also be high in calories, fats, sodium, or sugar.

Sugar Free

Sugar free doesn't mean a product has fewer calories than the regular version; it may have more. Sugar free products have less than 0.5 grams of sugar per serving by adding artificial sugar, but they still contain calories and carbohydrates from other sources.

Free Range

The USDA's definition for "Free Range" is that birds must have access to the outdoors. In some cases, this can mean access only through a hole in the wall or an open window, with no full-body access to the outdoors and no minimum space requirement. There are also no requirements for the amount of time spent outdoors.

Fat Free

This is a notoriously misleading label. Before choosing a fat-free food, make sure the product isn't loaded with sugar or additives, and that it is actually lower in calories than the regular version.

Made with Real Fruit

Products that claim to be made with real fruit may not contain very much at all, or none of the type pictured on the box. Check the label carefully.

Light

Light may mean that some food products contain 1/3 fewer calories or 50% less fat. All health claims are regulated by the FDA and USDA. When it comes to cooking oil, light refers to the color of the oil rather than the calorie content of the oil. There is no low calorie version of cooking oil.

Organic

While organic was once a bit like the term all natural—open to interpretation—that's no longer true. If a product has a USDA label that says organic, 95% or more of the ingredients must have been grown or processed without synthetic fertilizers or pesticides (among other standards). Remember that organic is not the same as healthy. Organic food can still contain a lot of sugar, fat, and calories.

FRUIT

Fruit is the world's natural, healthy sweet. Fruit contains sugar of course, but it also contains lots of fiber that fills you up quicker and satisfies your appetite and sweet tooth longer. Fruit metabolizes the natural sugar much slower and differently than processed sugars.

You can't compare all the benefits of real fruit to processed sweets, which have no benefits and lots of empty calories and fat; so highlight all the fruits you like from the list, but eliminate or limit your intake of very high carb fruits such as bananas, dates, and raisins.

How sweet and beautiful they are!

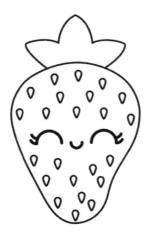

Apple

Apricot

Avocado

Banana

Black currant

Blackberry

Blueberry

Breadfruit

Cantaloupe

Carambola

Cherimoya

Cherry

Clementine

Coconut

Cranberry

Custard apple

Date

Durian

Elderberry

Feijoa

Fig fresh

Gooseberry

Grapefruit

Grape

Guava

Honeydew melon

Jackfruit

Java plum

Jujube

Kiwi

Kumquat

Lemon

Lime

Longan

Mango

Olive black

Olive Kalamata

Olive green

Orange

Papaya

Pear

Rose-apple

Sapodilla

Sapote

Soursop

Strawberry

Watermelon

Add any FRUIT not listed:

CHEESE

There are hundreds of types of cheese available in the world. Cheese calories range from 28 calories per oz. for cottage cheese to 291 per oz. for cream cheese.

Most cheeses are a good source of protein and calcium, and some offer additional health benefits. In particular, certain cheeses may provide nutrients that aid weight loss, improve bone health, and decrease your risk of heart disease. However, some types of cheese can be high in sodium and fat, so keep an eye on your intake.

American
Blue
Brie
Camembert
Cheddar
Cottage
Cream
Feta
Goat
Gouda
Mozzarella
Parmesan
Ricotta
Romano
String
Swiss

Add any CHEESE not listed:

MEAT

Do choose the least processed meats available, if you want. Cured and heavily processed meats such as lunch or deli meats contain a lot of salt, fat and sometimes sugar. Always choose quality when you can.

I list ground beef, but I don't advocate it. Most ground meat products contain lots of fat.

In order for ground meat to taste good and stay moist, it needs to have a percentage of animal fat added to it. Most ground meat offered at the market has between 20-40% added fat.

If you're going to eat ground meat, cook it, and remove most of the fat first, before you make a meal of it.

Bacon
Bison
Chicken
Duck
Goose
Ground beef
Ham
Lamb
Pork
Rabbit
Roast beef
Steak

Turkey
Venison
Wild boar

Add any MEAT not listed:

SEAFOOD

Anchovies
Barracuda
Basa
Bass
Black cod
Blowfish
Bluefish
Bream
Brill
Butter fish
Catfish
Clam
Cod
Crab
Crayfish
Cuttlefish
Dogfish
Dorado
Eel
Flounder
Grouper
Haddock
Hake
Halibut
Herring
Ilish

Lamprey
Langostine
Lingcod
Lobster
Mackerel
Mahi Mahi
Monkfish
Mullet
Mussel
Octopus
Orange roughie
Oyster
Perch
Pike
Pilchard
Pollock
Pomfret
Pompano
Sablefish
Salmon
Sanddab
Sardine
Scallop
Sea bass
Shad
Shark

Shrimp
Skate
Smelt
Snakehead
Snapper
Sole
Sprat
Squid
Sturgeon
Surimi
Swordfish
Tilapia
Tilefish
Trevally
Trout
Tuna
Turbot
Wahoo
Whitefish
Whiting

**Add any
SEAFOOD not
listed:**

VEGGIES want to be your friend. Embrace them.

If prepared the way you like, veggies can be very delicious.

Steam, sauté, bake or grill them.

Arrowroot	Chicory	Onion
Artichoke	Collard	Pepper banana
Arugala	Corn	Pepper green
Asparagus	Crookneck	Pepper red
Bamboo shoot	Cucumber	Pepper yellow
Beans green	Daikon	Pumpkin
Beet	Dandelion	Radicchio
Belgian endive	Edamame	Radish
Bitter melon	Eggplant	Rutabaga
Bok choy	Fennel	Salsify
Broad bean	Ginger	Shallot
Broccoli	Horseradish	Snow pea
Broccoli rabe	Jicama	Sorrel
Brussel sprout	Kale	Spinach
Cabbage green	Kohlrabi	Sugar snap pea
Cabbage red	Leek	Swiss chard
Cassava	Lettuce	Tomatillo
Cauliflower	Mustard Green	Tomato
Celeriac	Okra	**Add any**
Celery	Onion red	**VEGETABLE not**
Chayote	Onion green	**listed:**

STARCHY VEGETABLES are high in carbs
and calories, so use only 1/3 cup of them per day. Starchy
vegetables pack around 3–4 times more carbs than non-
starchy types. That's because they contain a similar number
of carbs as bread, rice, pasta and cereals.

Beans (black, kidney, navy, pinto, fava, cannellini)
Carrot
Chickpea
Corn
Lentil
Parsnip
Peas
Plantain
Potato red
Potato white
Potato yellow
Pumpkin
Squash winter
Squash acorn
Squash butternut
Squash spaghetti
Sweet potato
Taro
Yam

MUSHROOMS

Black Trumpet
Chanterelle
Cremini
Enoki
Maitake
Morel
Oyster
Porcini
Portobello
Shitake
White button

NUTS

Almond
Brazil nut
Cashew
Hazelnut
Macadamia
Peanut
Pecan
Pine nut
Pistachio
Walnut

Add any NUT not listed:

SEEDS

Chia

Add any SEED not listed:

Hemp

Pomegranate

Poppy

Pumpkin

Sesame

Sunflower

OIL

is pure FAT. 1 tbsp. = 119 calories. Use a little.

Avocado

Add any OIL not listed:

Canola

Coconut

Ghee

Grapeseed

Olive

Palm

Peanut

Safflower

Sesame

Sunflower

Walnut

ALCOHOLIC BEVERAGES

Alcohol can be enjoyed in moderation. In fact, dry wine has very few carbs and hard liquor none, but beer is fairly high in carbs.

And don't forget, that when we drink alcohol, we tend to eat and drink more than we need to.

BEVERAGES

BUTTER

is pure FAT. 1 tbsp. = 102 calories. Use a little.

CHEAT FOOD or maybe not

CHOCOLATE DARK

CONDIMENTS

DAIRY

EGGS

GRAINS (whole)

Even healthy, whole-grains are high in carbs and should be minimized. No more than 1/3 cup per day.

Barley

Buckwheat

Bulgur

Kasha

Quinoa

Oatmeal whole, rolled, or steel-cut

HERBS and SPICES

JELLY

Choose one with very low or no sugar

NUT BUTTERS

Choose one with no sugar

Almond

Cashew

Hazelnut

Peanut

PASTA

Italian

Cellophane noodles (mung bean)

Rice noodles

Soba noodles (buckwheat)

PASTA SAUCE

POPCORN

Choose one that is the least processed and low in calories, salt and no sugar.

RICE

I would not recommend white rice. It is highly processed. White rice increases blood sugar much more quickly than other types of rice. Try a whole grain rice instead.
Basmati
Black
Brown

Jasmine
Red
Wild

SWEETENERS

LOW-CARB TORTILLA
OR SLICE OF BREAD

Choose one that is 10 carbs and under.

YOGURT

Choose one that has little or no sugar.

_____

_____

_____

_____

_____

My Checklist

❏ I completed my Treat list

❏ I have all my kitchen items

❏ I selected and highlighted the foods I like on the #1 Acceptable Food List

❏ I chose my low-carb tortilla or bread product

❏ I chose my pasta sauce

❏ I carefully chose my condiments and listed them on the #1 Acceptable Food List

❏ I listed my favorite drinks

❏ I completed one drink comparison

❏ I designed my own menu using only the food items listed on the #1 Acceptable Food List

❏ I listed the processed foods I crave with their nutritional content

❏ I created my own food shopping list

❏ I purged all my processed foods from my home, car and place of work

❏ I shopped for real food

❏ I now eat and enjoy real foods

❏ I completed my booty shaker list

❏ I completed my gratitude list

❏ I completed my natural high list.

Made in the USA
Monee, IL
24 August 2021

75872984R00056